BLOOD TRANSFUSION

THINGS YOU SHOULD KNOW
(QUESTIONS AND ANSWERS)

By Rumi Michael Leigh

Introduction

I would like to thank and congratulate you for purchasing this book, " *Blood transfusion, things you should know (questions and answers)*" series.

This book will help you understand, revise and have a good general knowledge and keywords of Blood transfusion.

Thanks again for purchasing this book, I hope you enjoy it!

Chapter 1

1) What is a blood transfusion ?

   A blood transfusion is the transfer of new red blood cells to a patient through a vein.

2) What are some of the reasons of having a blood transfusion ?

- Some of the reasons of having a blood transfusion are an accident, surgery, cancers, renal failure, etc.

3) What are the signs of insufficient red blood cells ?

- The signs of insufficient red blood cells are fatigue, pale appearance, tachycardia, shortness of breath, etc.

4) What are some transfusion reactions ?

- Transfusion reactions include nausea, vomiting, chest pain, shortness of breath, sweating, itching, headache, etc.

5) What is a homologous transfusion ?

- A homologous transfusion is a transfusion by an anonymous donor.

6) What is an autologous transfusion ?

- An autologous transfusion is an autotransfusion (a recycling of a patient's own blood).

7) What is an allogenic transfusion ?

- An allogenic transfusion is a blood transfusion taken from another person.

8) What is the purpose of pre-transfusion testing ?

- The purpose of pre-transfusion testing is to avoid hemolytic transfusion reactions.

9) What is a genotype ?

- A genotype is a set of genes inherited by an individual.

10) What is a phenotype ?

- A phenotype consists of characteristics that can be observed in an individual.

Chapter 2

1) What are antigens ?

- Antigens are substances that can cause an immune reaction.

2) Where are antigens located ?

- Antigens surround the surface of red blood cells.

3) What is the function of antibodies ?

- Antibodies protect the body from antigens.

4) What is another name for antibodies ?

- Another name for antibodies is immunoglobulins.

5) What happens if there is the presence of the same antigen and the same antibody ?

- The presence of the same antigen and the same antibody will cause the destruction of red blood cells. The red blood cells will die.

6) What is agglutination ?

- Agglutination is the clumping of red blood cells that cause their death due to a blood group incompatibility with another blood group.

7) What is the cause of a hemolytic reaction ?

- A hemolytic reaction is a reaction that occurs due to the incompatibility between a patient's blood and a donor's blood.

8) Is a hemolytic reaction serious ?

- Yes, a hemolytic reaction is serious and can cause death.

9) What is an anaphylactic reaction ?

- An anaphylactic reaction is a life-threatening allergic reaction.

10) What is bronchoconstriction ?

- Bronchoconstriction is the narrowing of the airways in the lungs by the tightening of smooth muscles.

11) What is vasodilatation ?

- Vasodilatation is the widening of the blood vessels.

Chapter 3

1) What is plasma ?

-   Plasma is a substance in the blood that contains red blood cells, white blood cells and platelets.

2) What is the main function of the red blood cells ?

-   The main function of the red blood cells is the transport of oxygen.

3) What is the main function of the white blood cells?

-   The main function of the white blood cells is to fight against infections.

4) What are the functions of platelets ?

-   The function of platelets is blood clotting.

5) What are the effects of histamine ?

-   Histamine causes bronchoconstriction, vasodilation, and increased permeability of vessels.

6) What is tachycardia ?

-   Tachycardia is an abnormal rapid heartbeat.

7) What is tachypnea ?

- Tachypnea is an abnormal rapid breathing.

8) What is dyspnea ?

- Dyspnea is difficulty in breathing.

9) What is pruritus ?

- Pruritus is the sensation of itching on the skin.

10) What is oncotic pressure ?

- Oncotic pressure is a pressure that allows the retention of fluid.

11) What is the effect of proteins on oncotic pressure?

- Proteins increase oncotic pressure.

Chapter 4

1) What are the principal blood phenotypes ?

- The principal blood phenotypes are A, B, AB, and O.

2) What are the blood genotypes ?

- The blood genotypes are AA or AO, BB or BO, AB or OO.

3) What is the antigen of blood group A ?

- The antigen of blood group A is A.

4) What is the antigen of blood group B ?

- The antigen of blood group B is B.

5) What is the antigen of blood group AB ?

- The antigen of blood group AB is A and B.

6) What is the antigen of blood group O ?

- There is no antigen for blood group O.

7) What is the blood group A antibody ?

- The blood group A antibody is B antibody.

8) What is the blood group B antibody ?

- The blood group B antibody is A antibody.

9) What is the blood group AB antibody ?

- There is no antibody for blood group AB.

10) What is the blood group O antibody ?

- The blood group O antibody is the antibody A and the antibody B.

Chapter 5

1) What blood type is a universal recipient ?

- Blood type AB is a universal recipient.

2) Why is blood type AB a universal recipient ?

- Blood type AB is a universal recipient because it does not have any antibodies in the plasma.

3) Who can a person with a type O blood receive blood from ?

- A person with a type O blood can receive blood only from a person with type O blood.

4) Why is it that a person with a type O blood can only receive blood from another type O blood person ?

- A person with a type O blood can only receive blood from another type O blood person because of the presence of A and B antibodies in their blood.

5) Who can a person with type A blood receive blood from ?

- A person with type A blood can receive blood from a person with type A blood and type O blood.

6) Why can a person with type A blood receive blood from a person with type O blood ?

- A person with type A blood can receive blood from a person with type O blood because type O blood does not have B antigens.

7) Can a person with type A blood receive blood from a person with type B or type AB blood ?

- No, a person with type A blood cannot receive blood from a person with type B or type AB blood.

8) Why can't a person with type A blood receive blood from a person with type B or type AB blood?

- A person with type A blood cannot receive blood from a person with type B or type AB blood because they both have B antigens.

9) Who can a person with type A blood donate to ?

- A person with type A blood can donate to a person with type A and AB blood.

10) Can a person with type A blood donate to a person with type B blood ?

- No, a person with type A blood cannot donate to a person with type B blood.

Chapter 6

1) Why can't a person with type A blood donate to a person with type B blood ?

- A person with type A blood cannot donate to a person with type B blood because a person with type B blood has A antibodies.

2) Can a person with type A blood donate to a person with type O blood ?

- No, a person with type A blood cannot donate to a person with type O blood.

3) Why can't a person with type A blood donate to a person with type O blood ?

- A person with type A blood cannot donate to a person with type O blood because type O blood has A antibodies.

4) Why can a person with type A blood donate to a person with type AB blood ?

- A person with type A blood can donate to a person with type AB blood because a person with type AB blood does not have an A antibody.

5) Who can a person with type B blood receive blood from ?

- A person with type B blood can receive blood from a person with type B and type O blood.

6) Why can a person with type B blood receive blood from a person with type O blood ?

- A person with type B blood can receive blood from a person with type O blood because type O blood does not contain A antigen.

7) Why can't a person with type B blood receive blood from a person with type A and type AB blood ?

- A person with type B blood cannot receive blood from a person with type A and type AB blood because the person with type AB blood has an A antigen.

8) Who can a person with type B blood give blood to?

- A person with type B blood can give blood to a person with type B blood and type AB blood.

9) Why can a person with type B blood give blood to a person with type AB blood ?

- A person with type B blood can give blood to a person with type AB blood because a person with type AB blood does not have a B antibody.

10) Can a person with type B blood give blood to a person with type A and type O blood ?

- No, a person with type B blood cannot give blood to a person with type A and type O blood because a person with type A and type O blood have B antibodies.

Chapter 7

1) Who can a person with type AB blood receive blood from ?

- A person with type AB blood can receive blood from a person with type AB, A, B, and O blood. A person with type AB blood can receive blood from everybody.

2) Why can a person with type AB blood receive blood from everybody ?

- A person with type AB blood can receive blood from everybody because type AB blood does not have antibodies.

3) Who can a person with type AB blood give blood to ?

- A person with type AB blood can give blood to only a person with type AB blood.

4) Why can't a person with type AB blood give blood to a person with type A blood ?

- A person with type AB blood cannot give blood to a person with type A blood because type A blood has B antibodies.

5) Why can't a person with type AB blood give blood to a person with type B blood ?

- A person with type AB blood cannot give blood to a person with type B blood because type B blood has A antibodies.

6) Why can't a person with type AB blood give blood to a person with type O blood ?

- A person with type AB blood cannot give blood to a person with type O blood because type O blood has A and B antibodies.

7) Who can a person with type O blood receive blood from ?

- A person with type O blood can only receive blood from a person with type O blood.

8) Why can a person with type O blood only receive blood from a person with type O blood ?

- A person with type O blood can only receive blood from a person with type O blood because a person with type O blood has antibodies A and antibodies B.

9) Why can a person with type O blood give blood to everybody ?

- A person with type O blood can give blood to everybody because type O blood has no antigens.

10) What is the importance of the absence of antigens in type O blood as a universal donor ?

- The importance of the absence of antigens in type O blood as a universal donor is that the absence of antigens cannot provoke an immune response.

Chapter 8

1) What does the presence of a Rh factor on the surface of a blood cell signify ?

- The presence of a Rh factor on the surface of a blood cell signifies that it is Rh positive.

2) What does the absence of a Rh factor on the surface of a blood cell signify ?

- The absence of a Rh factor on the surface of a blood cell signifies that it is Rh negative.

3) What does the positive sign in Rhesus positive signify ?

- The positive sign in Rhesus positive signifies the presence of D antigen.

4) What does negative sign in Rhesus negative signify ?

- The negative sign in Rhesus negative signifies the absence of D antigen.

5) What is an AB positive ?

- An AB positive is the blood group AB with a Rh-positive factor.

6) What is an AB negative ?

- An AB negative is the blood group AB with a Rh-negative factor.

7) What is an A positive ?

- An A positive is the blood group A with a Rh-positive factor.

8) What is an A negative ?

- An A negative is the blood group A with a Rh-negative factor.

9) What is an O positive ?

- An O positive is the blood group O with a Rh-positive factor.

10) What is an O negative ?

- An O negative is the blood group O with a Rh-negative factor.

11) What kind of blood can a person with Rh positive factor receive ?

- A person with a Rh-positive factor can receive both Rh-positive and Rh-negative blood.

12) What kind of blood can a person with Rh-negative factor receive ?

- A person with a Rh-negative factor can only receive Rh-negative blood.

Chapter 9

1) What is the abbreviation TACO ?

- Transfusion-associated circulatory overload.

2) Is age a factor of risk for TACO ?

- Yes, age is a factor of risk for TACO.

3) What is the abbreviation GvHD ?

- Graft versus host disease.

4) What is the cause of GvHD ?

- GvHD is caused when a donor's bone marrow or stem cells recognize the patient's body as an invader, or a foreign body and attacks it.

5) When does GvHD usually occur ?

- GvHD usually occurs a couple of days or weeks after the transfusion.

6) What causes the immune response in a GvHD ?

- The T lymphocytes of the donor causes the immune response in a GvHD.

7) What is a gauge ?

- A gauge is the measure, size or capacity of an object.

8) What kind of gauge is necessary for an IV access during a transfusion ?

- A large gauge is necessary for an IV access during a transfusion.

9) Why is it important to use a large gauge during an IV transfusion ?

- It is important to use a large gauge during an IV transfusion because if the gauge is not large enough, the red blood cells can lysis.

10) Can an IV access used for a blood transfusion also be used for an intravenous drug ?

- No, an intravenous access used for a blood transfusion cannot be used for an intravenous drug, a second intravenous access is necessary.

Chapter 10

1) What is Septicemia ?

- Septicemia is a serious infection of the blood.

2) What kind of transfusion reaction is there a risk of jaundice ?

- There is a risk of jaundice in a hemolytic transfusion reaction.

3) What is febrile ?

- Febrile means signs and symptoms of fever.

4) What is the cause of a febrile reaction during transfusion ?

- A febrile reaction during transfusion is caused when the patient's white blood cells react with the donor's white blood cells that then causes an increase in temperature.

5) What solution is used when transfusing blood ?

- When transfusing blood, a saline 0.9% is used.

6) When is a blood warmer usually used during a transfusion ?

- A blood warmer is usually used during a transfusion when a patient needs rapidly large amounts of blood transfusion.

7) What is the function of fluids in a transfusion reaction ?

- Fluids help the body get rid of free hemoglobin.

8) What is free hemoglobin ?

- Free hemoglobin is the hemoglobin that is outside of the red blood cells.

9) What is TRALI ?

- Translated acute lung injury.

10) What could be noticed in a patient's blood who has had frequent blood transfusions ?

- A patient who has had frequent blood transfusions have high iron levels in the blood.

Chapter 11

1) What is a disseminated intravascular coagulation?

- A disseminated intravascular coagulation is a disorder which causes the formation of blood clots throughout the body, blocking small blood vessels.

2) What is the first thing to do if a patient has a transfusion reaction ?

- The first thing to do if a patient has a transfusion reaction is to stop the transfusion and replace it with NaCl 0.9%.

3) What are the types of medications administered during a transfusion reaction ?

- Antihistamines, vasopressors, corticosteroids, antipyretics, diuretics, fluids, etc. are some types of medications administered during a transfusion reaction.

4) What are vasopressors ?

- Vasopressors are drugs that cause vasoconstriction.

5) What are the functions of corticosteroids in a transfusion reaction ?

- Corticosteroids is anti-inflammatory and suppresses the immune system activity.

6) What kind of patients can have a circulatory overload during a transfusion ?

- Patients with renal failure or patients with congestive heart failure can have a circulatory overload during a transfusion.

Conclusion

Thank you again for purchasing this book. I hope it has helped you in your journey to understanding Blood transfusion.

Thank you.